Depression

How a woman can fight depression and get her life back

Melissa Keane

Introduction

I would like to thank you for downloading the book, *"Depression"*.

This book has actionable information on how to fight depression as a woman.

Depression is a serious condition that affects everyone; however, as research has shown, women are twice as likely to experience stress, anxiety, and depression.

This book solely focuses on depression in women: why it happens, its symptoms and how to ease it and all its latent signs and symptoms. This book teaches you ways through which to ease stress and anxiety and cure depression without reliance on medicine and extensive medical treatments.

It is important to remember that depression is treatable; because you are depressed right now (or experience rampant depression every so often) does not mean depression is there to stay. By reading this book, you will learn simple ways to eliminate depression from your life using natural treatments and lifestyle changes.

Thank you again for downloading this book. I hope you enjoy it!

Best,

Melissa Keane

Health Secrets for Her

Table of Contents

What Causes Depression In Women

Depression is a condition taken lightly by many; thus, it goes untreated and continues wreaking lives. As stated earlier, women are 50% more likely to suffer from depression, which means as a woman, your chances of suffering from this condition are high.

However, to prevent the onset of depression, or to cure it if you are suffering from it, you first need to understand depression; after all, is it not true that, *"To acquire knowledge, one must study; but to acquire wisdom, one must observe?"* - **Marilyn vos Savant**

Thus, to overcome depression, we first must cultivate a clear understanding of it. Let us do that now:

Understanding Depression

Depression refers instances where you are feeling sad, discouraged, stressed, hopeless, uninterested, and unmotivated for considerably long periods. Feeling extremely low and gloomy is normal when you go through a bad episode such as losing a loved one or an important job.

However, if you let these feelings overstay their welcome, say for instance, for more than two weeks, and allow them to take over your mind, this can easily lead to depression.

When you allow a negative feeling to dwell in your mind for long, it slowly starts interfering with your normal thinking process. You start to think under the shadows of that negative thought and continue ruminating on it.

For instance, if your spouse cheated on you and divorced you saying you are not deserving of him, instead of moving on with your life after brief sadness and grief, you let those negative thoughts stick and you stay gloomy 24/7.

You let those negative thoughts live in your mind and soon, they corrupt your normal thinking. Whenever you cannot do something right, you think it happened because you are not good enough. You start becoming stressed and when this behavior continues for more than two to three weeks, it turns into depression.

To gain full understanding of depression, it is important to be aware of its causes so you understand what triggers the condition:

Causes Of Depression

Depression has many causes/triggers; therefore, it is important to know each of them so you can self-diagnose yourself and be on your way to recovery.

Below are major causes of depression in women:

Premenstrual Dysphoric Disorder (PMDD)

PMDD is a condition that affects 3-8% of menstruating females; PMDD is a severe form of Premenstrual Stress (PMS). PMDD is also a depressive disorder that causes you to feel irritable, tired, anxious, and helpless.

The symptoms, on average, start six days before your menstruation cycle begins and end almost as soon as they begin. However, the symptoms can also last for two weeks and are worse two days before you start menstruating.

The cause of PMS and PMDD is the hormonal fluctuation you go through during a menstrual cycle. The three hormones that control the menstrual cycle are progesterone, estrogen, and testosterone.

Estrogen controls your emotions; its levels are relatively low before and during the first few days of your period. Once you start menstruating, you feel better after the first day or two because of a surge of estrogen in the brain.

The problem with PMDD is that it is so much more than a normal mood disorder. The hormonal fluctuations enhance the effects of any coexisting mood disorders, which then spin your emotions out of control.

For instance, if you are battling with stress and anxiety, when you are menstruating, you are likely to be more stressed and anxious, which can easily lead to depression.

Postpartum Depression

Most women only feel depressive in the first few weeks, but if the depression persists for months and becomes severe, it turns into postpartum depression.

When a woman is pregnant, her progesterone and estrogen levels are high, but after birth, levels of these hormones considerably drop causing hormonal fluctuations. Moreover, the overwhelming feeling of taking care of a child paired with the exhaustion and sleeplessness worsens postpartum depression.

It is important to point out that experiencing a little depression after having your baby is normal; however, if you feel depressed all the time, not enjoying your baby's coos and little movements, you could be suffering from postpartum depression. This may happen when you continuously think of the difficult phase you went through as you carried your baby to term and birth.

In addition, postpartum depression may strike women who did not want to have a baby in the first place or who bear the responsibility of nurturing the child (for instance, single mothers with no one to rely on for support).

For instance, Liby (name changed) suffered from postpartum depression at the age of 25 after having her first child. She wanted a baby, but her partner did not; so, he broke up with her and she had to bear the huge responsibility alone. Although she got counseling three months after having her baby, the first three months of caring for the child were terrible for her.

Infertility

Women suffering from infertility are at a high risk of developing depression because they are emotionally vulnerable. Women are naturally born to nurture and they best do this by taking care of a child. Therefore, not being able to conceive can lead to feelings of anger, guilt, and sadness because motherhood is dear to every woman.

Moreover, the medication used to treat infertility causes depression because it alters your hormones. For example, to improve ovulation in women, doctors prescribe Clomid or Serophene (synthetic estrogen clomiphene citrate). These medications have the side effects of causing anxiety, sleep interruption, and depression.

Stress

One of the psychological causes of depression in women is stress. The stress could be home or work related. Such depression is more prevalent in women because their physiological response to stress varies from that in men.

Unlike men, women produce more stress hormones such as Corticoliberin or CRF. Our bodies also produce progesterone; progesterone keeps the stress hormone in the body active (it keeps it from automatically switching off).

Rumination

Rumination is a psychological cause of depression in women. This study shows that unlike men, who when depressed, distract themselves, women are more likely to discuss feelings with friends, try to figure out the cause of the depression, or cry to assuage latent feelings of depression and stress.

Whenever we feel depressed, we ruminate on bad memories; this rumination causes a transient episode of depression to prolong its stay and turn it into severe depression.

Now that you are well aware of what may cause depression in women, let us discuss what you can do about it.

How To Treat Depression

In the subsequent chapters, we are going to look at different natural ways to treat depression.

Identify The Symptoms

When I was first depressed, I did not understand my condition until it had spread its roots deep into my life. I lost my job and cancer took my best friend one month after losing my job.

When these things happened, one after the other, I started losing hope and slowly started succumbing to depression. I began with giving up on finding good jobs and then started shutting myself off from loved ones. I munched on comfort foods and gained about 20 pounds in three months. Although I just thought I was going through a rough patch and trying to cope, my mother pointed out that I could be depressed and hearing depression as this big scary word, I did not want to suffer from the condition any longer; thus, I made a decision to do something about my life.

By making me look for, and understand its symptom, my mother helped me understand depression and its adverse effects on my life. If you fear you are going through depression, the first step is to look for its symptoms.

After you are sure the condition has afflicted you, only then can you embark on the journey to overcoming it using the techniques I used, and millions of women across the globe have used to overcome depression.

Symptoms Of Depression

Depression has several noticeable symptoms that make it easier to diagnose yourself if you closely monitor yourself. Here are the symptoms you should be on the lookout for:

Persistent Sadness

Common symptoms of depression include feeling persistently sad for weeks, months, or even years. However, do not make the mistake of confusing sadness that lasts a few hours as a symptom of depression. If you are suffering from depression, you will feel low and sad on a regular and consistent basis.

The sadness persists because instead of focusing on the person or issue causing the sadness, we are often quick to heap blame on ourselves. Moreover, if the cause of the sadness is a spouse, he may react by blaming you because that is how men react when depressed; this only adds to your depression.

Hopelessness and Helplessness

Feeling hopeless simply means feeling as if life has no meaning and nothing good can happen to you. Moreover, when you feel hopeless and helpless, you feel incapable of controlling anything in life or as if there is nothing you can do to improve your situation.

Loss of Interest

Another noticeable symptom of depression is losing all interest in hobbies, pastimes, activities, work, and social life. Moreover, if you are depressed, you will feel as if you have lost the ability to feel joy or pleasure.

Changes in Sleep Pattern

While other reasons such as sleep apnea could account for changes in your sleep pattern, a sudden change in your sleep pattern could also be due to depression. A change in sleep pattern means you will feel either extremely sleepy or not sleepy at all which results in insomnia.

From personal experience, women tend to sleep less when depressed because they stay up and ponder over the mishaps in their life. For instance, when I went through my depressed period, I slept for 12 hours straight daily for about two months. Yes, I know it is a bit too much but I did not have anything else to do (at least that is what I thought).

Changes in Weight

A sudden change in weight, such as becoming excessively overweight or becoming extremely underweight, could be a sign of depression. If you feel you have lost your appetite, or you feel a considerable increase in your appetite within a matter days, then you may be suffering from depression.

Men generally rely more on alcohol and drugs as avenues for dealing with depression; women, on the other hand, rely on comfort food (ice cream, chocolate); this can lead to a weight increase. However, in severe cases of depression, you can completely lose your appetite, which leads to weight loss. In my case, my appetite increased.

Loss of Energy

Loss of energy is another depression symptom you should look out for; for instance, if you start feeling fatigued without an increase in physical activity, then depression could be the reason. Loss of energy can also include feeling sluggish or physically drained all the time.

Self-Hatred

Another common symptom of depression in women is feeling an extreme sense of hatred towards yourself. For instance, feeling worthless, feeling incapable of doing anything right or criticizing yourself over everything are all signs of self-hatred.

I find this feeling relatable because when I was depressed, I loathed myself.

Anger and Irritability

If you have been feeling unusually angry or irritable, this could be indicative of depression. When you are suffering from depression, you experience sudden outburst of anger and the smallest of things can infuriate you. If you are a reasonable and calm person, but you have started experiencing temper problems, you may be suffering from depression.

Persistent Physical Symptoms

If you are suffering from consistent headaches, upset stomach and pain despite taking medication for these conditions, depression might be the reason behind these sudden physical problems.

Suicidal Thoughts and Tendencies

If you are suffering from a severe form of depression, you may develop suicidal thoughts. Suicidal thoughts include thoughts about hurting yourself. This is depression's most dangerous symptom. Women are more prone to suicidal thoughts because they are more sensitive than men are.

Go through these symptoms again and observe yourself closely; use them to determine if you may be depressed. If you notice even a single one of these signs, if you do not take action immediately, the problem may exacerbate to critical levels.

Use NLP Techniques To Cure Depression

After determining you are a victim of this condition, swiftly move to treating it. One of the best ways to cure depression is using NLP techniques.

NLP stands for **Neuro-Linguistic Programming.** NLP is a behavioral technology that helps you change your current thought process, how you view your past, and how you deal with life and its many vicissitudes. NLP techniques are potent and powerful ways to take control of your mind. In step 2, we will discuss four of these techniques to help you overcome your depression.

Although you may find the term Neuro-Linguistic Programming intimidating, once I explain the simple NLP techniques you can use to cure depression, you will see NLP for what it is: an easy way to reprogram your mind and its language.

1st Technique: Reframing

Reframing is an interesting NLP technique ideally suited to curing depression. Reframing simply means putting a different spin on a situation and seeing it in a different light.

For instance, when you are experiencing a depressive episode because of an argument that has distanced you from your spouse, put a different spin on the situation by thinking 'maybe this fight will bring us closer because it gave us a chance to express ourselves and opinions.' You can follow a simple six-step framework to find the positive intention behind a bad or unwanted behavior.

1. When reframing, the first thing to do is identify an unwanted behavior. Assume the behavior you want to change is negative self-talk.

2. Next, communicate with the part of your body responsible for this unwanted behavior. In this case, the part of your body you will communicate to is your brain because that is where the negative self-talk births. When your brain responds to your signal, acknowledge it and thank it.

3. Now, identify the positive intention behind your behavior by asking yourself what positive outcome it aims to achieve through negative self-talk. For instance, the positive intention of your brain behind negative self-talk could be to remind you of your mistakes so you do not repeat them in the future.

4. Once you identify the positive intention, ask your mind to create three new behaviors that could yield results similar to your previous behavior. For instance, to remind yourself of your mistake you could practice positive self-talk and use affirmations.

5. Next, ask your brain to evaluate the new behaviors and tell you if it is willing to accept them. Once your brain accepts the new behaviors, you will feel it in your body and if you do not, repeat step four until you feel the acceptance.

6. Finally, ask other parts of your body if they will work in unison with your brain on the new behaviors and make sure there is no disagreement.

This technique greatly helps you eliminate any unwanted behaviors that cause depression.

2nd Technique: Memory Manipulation

Another NLP technique usable to cure depression is Memory Manipulation. Memory manipulation helps you alter how you feel about a certain memory. You can practice this technique by following these simple steps.

1. Pick a memory you want to change and feel differently about, perhaps a memory that causes depression. The memory has to be about something that makes you sad every time you think about it. For instance, the memory could be failing a job interview you really wanted to pass because you saw it as the only opportunity to move forward in life.

Once you have pinpointed the memory you want to change, (in this case, a failed interview), your mind will play a reel full of images of that memory; soon, you will feel various negative emotions rushing in inside you.

2. Now, you have to stop the reel and pick a single image to represent the memory of your failed interview. Once the image is in front of you, step back from your memory and look at it from an outsider's point of view.

3. Now, play with this memory by placing a frame around it and analyze if doing this has made the feeling less intense. Make the picture black and white, make it blurry, take it out of focus, and determine how these changes make you feel; the purpose of this exercise is to dissociate from the negative memory.

4. If the third step yields little progress, put a humorous spin on your memory. For instance, put a wig or a clown face on the person interviewing you. Try to smile or laugh as you make these changes.

5. Next, play with the sounds in your memory. For instance, slow down or increase the pace at which the interviewer is asking you questions. You can also make the voice louder or quieter and determine which one makes you feel better.

If an insult from the interviewer or the words he or she used to reject you are the ones hurting you the most, then change the voice of that person and assume it was that of a funny cartoon character such as Donald Duck. It is impossible to take someone seriously when he or she is mimicking Donald Duck.

This exercise will help you determine which changes to your memory lessen the negative feelings attached to it. You can practice this technique on several other memories that make you feel depressed. Next time you practice Memory Manipulation, take a harsher memory, and apply these steps to it until the memory no longer haunts you.

3rd Technique: Collapsing Anchors

Collapsing Anchors is another powerful NLP technique used to eliminate depressive feelings and emotions. To eliminate a negative state such as an encounter with a best friend who betrayed you, then collapsing anchors is the technique to practice.

This technique is one of the most useful NLP techniques you can use to cure depression because it eliminates negative factors causing your depression, and replaces it with feelings of happiness, confidence, and relief.

Practicing this technique will take 10 to 15 minutes after which, you will feel happier and stronger. Here is how to practice this technique:

1. When collapsing anchors, the first thing to do is identify the negative state you want to collapse. Choose a particular memory that causes depression; for instance, the end of a long friendship due to your friend's betrayal.

Once you have identified the negative state, choose a positive state you would like to use to override that negative state. For instance, think of a memory where you are happy and relaxed.

Just as you picked a specific negative memory, pick a specific time and place when you were in a positive state. For instance, the happiness, joy, and excitement you felt the first time you met your husband. It is important to note that for this technique to work; your positive memory or state should be more powerful than your negative state.

2. The next step is to set anchors. Setting anchors simply means associating a memory with a body gesture or movement. You can anchor the negative state to rubbing your left thumb and index finger together and reliving the negative memory.

Make sure you completely immerse in your memory and you can feel, hear, and see everything from your own eyes as it happened. Let your emotions reach their peak and break the anchor by rubbing your thumb and index finger together.

For the next 30 seconds, do something else to break the state and relax; you can do things such as sing, dance, skip, jump or scream. What you do is completely up to you. Repeat rubbing your left thumb and index finger; if the negative state starts to reappear, it means you have successfully anchored it.

3. This is the fun step of this technique because now you get to anchor your positive state. Do this by reliving your happy memory and completely immersing yourself in it, making it brighter, more colorful, and vivid. Anchor this state by rubbing the right thumb to your right index finger. When your emotions are at their peak, break the state and do something else for the next 30 seconds as you did in the previous step.

Like when anchoring the negative state, you have to anchor the positive state using either the same or the new positive memories repeatedly. Make sure you enjoy yourself each time you relive a positive memory because that is going to make it stronger. After practicing this step several times, rub your right thumb against the right index finger to see if you feel the positive memories rush back. If they do, then you have successfully anchored the positive state as well.

4. Now, collapse the two anchors. Start by rubbing your thumbs and index fingers of both hands together. In the next 30 seconds to 2 minutes, you may feel a bit confused because the two states will have started to integrate. Soon the positive state will start to override the negative state and you will feel a burst of positive emotions. Once you feel happy and relaxed, it means the anchors have collapsed. To be on the safe side, hold the anchors for another 10-15 seconds to ensure they have perfectly collapsed.

You can use different negative states that are the recurrent causes of your depression and collapse them with your happy memories in this manner. Soon, your depression will start decreasing because the causes will be eliminated one by one.

4th Technique: Pattern Interrupt

Pattern interrupt is an NLP technique used to stop a thought, action, behavior, or situation. It is a very useful technique to treat depression because it can stop a thought before it begins; meaning it cures depression by extracting it from its roots.

For example, if you practice negative self-talk on a regular basis, using pattern interrupt can eliminate your harsh self-talk before it starts.

Pattern interrupt is one of the easiest NLP techniques; you can master it with minimal practice. To practice pattern interrupt, simply start interrupting behaviors that push you into deep depression.

For instance, if you are in the habit of crying every time you feel a little sad, then start interrupting this pattern by introducing a new pattern to replace the crying. It is important to note that the interruption in the previous pattern i.e. crying should come as early as possible such as when you feel the urge to cry or the moment your first tear appears. Next time you want to cry, start jumping up and down, or start doing squats.

This might sound silly, but this actually works. To see its effectiveness, try it for the next few days. All you have to do is interrupt your crying by doing squats or anything that breaks the process and repeat this step until the previous pattern is no more.

Start working on these four wonderful NLP techniques and soon you will become happier and bid farewell to depression for good.

Make Lifestyle Changes To Cure Depression

Lifestyle changes are the best way to cure depression because by making lifestyle changes, you keep yourself from resorting to medication or therapy to cure depression. It is important to note that the healthier your body and mind are, the easier it will be to fight depression.

As soon as the first wave of depression hits, the first thing you are likely to do is indulge in a big bowl of ice cream or eat calorie rich hamburgers in attempts to shove your depressive feelings back with food.

In addition to resorting to eating heaps of fattening foods, you also start to become lazy and sedentary. Studies show that a sedentary and unhealthy lifestyle directly links to depression. The more inactive you are, the greater your chances of experiencing depression.

An inactive lifestyle causes you to neglect your health and make bad choices regarding your diet, drug use, exercise, and routine. When this happens, it is natural for your body and mind to be more prone to weakness.

Always remember that a weak mind cannot cultivate a positive attitude: the very thing you need to cure depression. To cure your depression for good, you must make healthy lifestyle changes.

Here are the various lifestyle changes you should implement to strengthen your mind and body to cure your depression.

Exercise

Exercising stimulates the brain into releasing feel good chemicals. These chemicals, known collectively as neurotransmitters include endorphins, dopamine, norepinephrine, and serotonin.

Regular exercise elevates the level of serotonin in your brain. This elevates your mood. Duke University conducted a study to show how exercising 30 minutes a day for four months can alleviate depression without resorting to medication.

Research also shows that aerobic exercises are the most effective at easing depression. These types of exercises elevate your heart rate, which then allows for better circulation in the brain, which in turn balances the chemicals in your brain.

Aerobic exercises can include brisk walking, jogging, cycling, swimming, and aerobic dancing. You can commit to any one of these you feel most comfortable doing.

By exercising regularly, you also benefit from the 'runner's high' which refers to feeling euphoric after a workout or run. The runner's high is a result of your body releasing endorphins when you exercise. Because they interact with the opiate receptors in the brain to reduce your perception of pain, endorphins act in a way similar to how morphine works.

A study shows women can benefit from endorphins more than men can because women already have higher levels of endorphins in their system and hence, they can achieve the runner's high with lesser effort.

To get the full benefits of exercise, you should develop an exercise routine by doing the following:

1. Jog every day for at least 15 minutes.

2. When you exercise, focus on your body movements because that will distract you from negative or upsetting thoughts.

3. Set exercise goals because achieving them will give you a sense of accomplishment, which will boost your mood. For instance, you can challenge yourself to do 30 squats twice a day for the next month.

4. If you have trouble committing to exercising, join an exercise class because it will help you stick to a schedule and allow you to meet new people.

By following this simple routine, you can begin to cure your depression.

Eat Healthy

You may not be aware of this, but what you eat affects how you feel because a nutritious diet protects your mental health and encourages physical fitness.

Women turn to food likes chocolate, ice cream, macaroni and cheese, French fries and fried chicken to relieve depression. These foods instigate a form of euphoric high that keeps away the dreaded return of depression. This effect comes about because high levels of sugar or lack of nutrients disrupts your bodily functions and you end up feeling worse than before.

To make your diet healthy and nutritious, do the following:

Eat More Magnesium: Magnesium helps the brain produce more serotonin, a hormone that improves your mood and makes you energetic. Women have low levels of magnesium than men; therefore, it is important to eat foods that contain magnesium. These foods include fish, sunflower, and pumpkin seeds, nuts, raw spinach, avocado, and brown rice.

Complex Carbohydrates: Adding complex carbohydrates such as whole-grain foods, sweet potatoes, legumes, beans, carrots and oats to your diet can lower levels of depression.

Complex carbohydrates are different from simple carbohydrates (simple sugars, white pasta, and white bread) because they lower your blood sugar whereas simple carbohydrates considerably increase blood sugar levels because your body breaks down simple carbohydrates much faster and complex carbohydrates take longer to break down leading to sugar highs and crashes.

Omega-3 Foods: A Norwegian study shows that regular intake of foods rich in omega-3 can reduce risk of depression by 30%. Another study shows that omega-3 can also help those already suffering from depression because women suffering from depression have low levels of chemicals called eicosapentaenoic acid (EPA) and docosahexaenoic acid (DHA) especially during pregnancy.

To increase omega-3 in your diet, eat foods such as sardines, tuna, walnuts, flax and chia seeds, wild salmon, egg yolk, and anchovies.

By making these simple yet necessary changes to your diet, you can cure depression.

Other Lifestyle Changes

Now that we have discussed the most important lifestyle changes you need to make to cure depression, let us discuss the other lifestyle changes you can make to cure depression.

Stay Hydrated: 85% of your brain is water; if you are dehydrated; you can feel irritable, lack focus, and feel a loss of energy making you more susceptible to stress, anxiety, and finally depression. Drink at least eight to ten glasses of water every day to stay fresh and hydrated.

Avoid Caffeine: Caffeine can increase and prolong depression. Various studies show the relation between high caffeine intake and increased depression.

If your caffeinated beverage intake is high, gradually minimize your consumption because quitting cold turkey results in side effects such as headaches and dizziness. Moreover, making a gradual shift helps you stay committed to your mission.

Sleep Well: Evidence suggests a lack of sleep can also lead to depression. If you are sleeping less than seven to eight hours a day, perhaps due to work or home related issues, start sleeping at least 8 hours every night. In addition, sleep in a quiet room that makes it easier to sleep peacefully and calmly.

Increase Vitamin Intake: Vitamins such as vitamin C, D and B are good for mental health; adding them to your daily diet is a good way to manage depression. In addition, it is important to note that sometimes, the cause of depression can be a lack of one of these vitamins in your body; hence, intake of vitamins eliminates depression.

Meditation: Last but not the least, make mindfulness meditation a regular practice because it helps alleviate depression.

To practice mindfulness, sit in a quiet area on a straight-backed chair or on the floor and if on the floor, cross your legs; if on a chair, ensure your feet touch the ground. Once seated, focus on how your body moves with your breathing movements. When your focus is solely on your breathing, allow your mind to wander and observe your thoughts as they pass. If you get distracted, re-focus on the breathing movements. The important thing is to observe thoughts without judging them.

Mindfulness meditation helps slow down your thought process so your thoughts flow in and out in a slow manner. When your thoughts enter and exit your mind in a calm manner, it becomes easier to spot them and differentiate between negative and positive thoughts.

As the identification of unhealthy thoughts becomes easier, you quickly spot a depression triggering thought and let it flow out of your mind easily without holding onto it. This practice helps you rid yourself of unhealthy thoughts and become strong enough to fight depression every time it starts to creep in your life.

Once you start implementing these lifestyle changes, you will experience a positive impact on your attitude and you will have the necessary mental strength to fight depression.

Conclusion

Thank you again for purchasing this book!

I hope this book was able to help you to know how you can deal with depression as a woman.

The next step is to use the information in this book to treat your depression.

Finally, if you enjoyed this book, would you be kind enough to leave a review for this book on Amazon?

Thank you and good luck!

Melissa Keane